THE COMPLETE LAMICTAL (LAMOTRIGINE) MEN USAGE MANUAL

Brasian Mone

© 2024 Brasian Mone. All rights reserved.

Disclaimer

The data gave on this stage is to instructive and educational purposes as it were. It isn't expected as a substitute for proficient clinical counsel, conclusion, or treatment. Continuously look for the counsel of your doctor or other qualified wellbeing supplier with any inquiries you might have in regards to an ailment. Never ignore proficient clinical guidance or postpone in looking for it in light of something you have perused on this stage.

Contents

CHAPTER ONE 1

Introduction 1

CHAPTER TWO 5

Uses 5

CHAPTER THREE 8

Side effects 8

CHAPTER FOUR 12

Interaction 12

CHAPTER FIVE 15

Dosages 15

CHAPTER SIX 23

FAQ 23

CHAPTER ONE

Introduction

Lamictal (lamotrigine) is an anticonvulsant medication primarily used to treat epilepsy and bipolar disorder. Its unique mechanism of action involves stabilizing neuronal membranes and inhibiting the release of excitatory neurotransmitters, which helps prevent seizures and mood episodes.

Indications:

Epilepsy: Lamictal is effective for both partial seizures and generalized seizures, making it suitable for a wide range of epilepsy types.

Bipolar Disorder: It is particularly noted for its efficacy in managing the depressive episodes associated with bipolar disorder and can help stabilize mood in patients experiencing rapid cycling.

Dosage and Administration:

Lamictal is available in various forms, including tablets, chewable tablets, and orally disintegrating tablets. Dosing typically begins at a low level to minimize the risk of skin rashes, particularly the serious condition known as Stevens-Johnson syndrome. The dosage is gradually increased based on the patient's response and tolerance.

Side Effects:

While many patients tolerate Lamictal well, some may experience side effects, which can include:

- **Common Side Effects**: Headache, dizziness, drowsiness, nausea, and insomnia.
- **Serious Side Effects**: Rash (which may progress to a more serious condition), fever, swollen lymph nodes, and unusual bruising

or bleeding. Regular monitoring for these symptoms is crucial, especially after the dosage is increased.

Drug Interactions:

Lamictal can interact with several other medications, affecting its metabolism. Drugs that induce liver enzymes (like some oral contraceptives or certain antiepileptic drugs) can lower Lamictal levels, while drugs that inhibit liver enzymes can raise its levels, increasing the risk of side effects.

Monitoring:

Patients on Lamictal should be regularly monitored, especially during the initial phase of treatment or when dosages are adjusted. Blood tests might be necessary to check for potential adverse effects or to ensure therapeutic levels are achieved.

Patient Considerations:

Pregnancy and Breastfeeding: Lamictal can be used during pregnancy, but it's essential to weigh the benefits against potential risks. It is also excreted in breast milk, so mothers should consult healthcare providers.

Withdrawal: Abruptly stopping Lamictal can lead to increased seizure frequency. Any changes in medication should be guided by a healthcare provider.

Lamictal is a vital option in the management of epilepsy and bipolar disorder, offering significant benefits for many patients. As with any medication, it requires careful management and monitoring to optimize therapeutic outcomes while minimizing risks. Always consult a healthcare provider for personalized advice and guidance when considering or using Lamictal.

CHAPTER TWO

Uses

Lamictal (lamotrigine) is primarily used for the following conditions:

Epilepsy:

- **Partial Seizures**: Effective for adults and children with partial seizures (focal seizures) that may or may not evolve into generalized seizures.
- **Generalized Seizures**: Used for various generalized seizure types, including tonic-clonic seizures and seizures associated with Lennox-Gastaut syndrome.

Bipolar Disorder:

- **Depressive Episodes**: Helps stabilize mood and is particularly effective in managing depressive episodes in individuals with bipolar disorder.

- **Maintenance Therapy**: Can be used to prevent mood episodes (both depressive and manic) in individuals with a history of bipolar disorder.

Off-Label Uses:

- **Anxiety Disorders**: Sometimes prescribed off-label for certain anxiety disorders, though this is less common.
- **Borderline Personality Disorder**: May be used to help manage emotional dysregulation in some patients.
- **Trigeminal Neuralgia**: In some cases, Lamictal may be used for nerve pain associated with trigeminal neuralgia.

Lamictal is a versatile medication that plays a crucial role in treating epilepsy and bipolar disorder, making it an essential tool in neurology and psychiatry. Always consult a healthcare professional for advice tailored to individual needs.

CHAPTER THREE

Side effects

Lamictal (lamotrigine) can cause a range of side effects, which may vary in severity. It's important to monitor for these effects, especially when starting treatment or adjusting the dosage. Here's a breakdown of potential side effects:

Common Side Effects:

- **Dizziness**: Lightheadedness or a feeling of being unsteady.
- **Headache**: May occur, particularly when starting the medication or increasing the dose.
- **Nausea**: Some patients may experience gastrointestinal discomfort.
- **Drowsiness**: Fatigue or sedation can occur, affecting daily activities.

- **Insomnia**: Difficulty sleeping may be reported by some individuals.
- **Rash**: A mild skin rash can develop; it's essential to monitor for more severe reactions.

Serious Side Effects:

- **Severe Skin Reactions**: Rash that can progress to Stevens-Johnson syndrome (SJS) or toxic epidermal necrolysis (TEN), both of which are life-threatening. Symptoms may include blistering, peeling skin, and flu-like symptoms. Immediate medical attention is required if a rash develops.
- **Aseptic Meningitis**: In rare cases, Lamictal can cause symptoms such as fever, headache, stiff neck, and sensitivity to light.
- **Blood Disorders**: Rarely, Lamictal may lead to conditions like leukopenia (low white blood cell count) or thrombocytopenia

(low platelet count), which can increase the risk of infections or bleeding.
- **Mood Changes**: Some patients may experience worsening depression or suicidal thoughts. Monitoring for mood changes is essential.

Other Considerations:

- **Withdrawal Symptoms**: Abruptly stopping Lamictal can lead to increased seizure frequency or withdrawal symptoms. Dosage changes should always be done under medical supervision.
- **Interactions with Other Medications**: Certain drugs can affect Lamictal's levels in the body, leading to increased side effects or decreased efficacy.

While many individuals tolerate Lamictal well, it's crucial to be aware of both common and serious side effects. Regular communication with a healthcare provider is important for monitoring and managing any adverse effects. If you experience any severe or unusual symptoms, seek medical attention promptly.

CHAPTER FOUR

Interaction

Lamictal (lamotrigine) can interact with various medications, which may affect its effectiveness or increase the risk of side effects. Here are some key interactions to be aware of:

Other Antiepileptic Drugs:

- **Inducers** (e.g., carbamazepine, phenytoin, phenobarbital): These can lower Lamictal levels, potentially leading to inadequate seizure control.
- **Inhibitors** (e.g., valproate): These can increase Lamictal levels, raising the risk of side effects, including serious skin reactions.

Hormonal Contraceptives:

- Certain hormonal contraceptives (like some birth control pills) can reduce Lamictal levels, potentially leading to breakthrough seizures. Adjustments in Lamictal dosage may be needed.

Medications for HIV:

- Drugs such as ritonavir or efavirenz can affect Lamictal metabolism, either increasing or decreasing its levels.

Other Medications:

- **Antidepressants**: Some may interact, though the specifics depend on the particular drug.
- **Antipsychotics**: There can be interactions with certain antipsychotic medications, affecting levels of either medication.

Alcohol:

- Alcohol can exacerbate drowsiness and dizziness, increasing the risk of side effects.

Monitoring and Consultation:

It's crucial for individuals taking Lamictal to inform their healthcare providers about all medications they are using, including over-the-counter drugs, supplements, and herbal products. Regular monitoring may be necessary when starting or stopping other medications.

If you have specific medications in mind or need more details about particular interactions, feel free to ask!

CHAPTER FIVE

Dosages

Lamictal (lamotrigine) dosages can vary depending on the condition being treated, the patient's age, and whether they are taking other medications. Here's a general overview of dosages:

Epilepsy:

Adults and Children Over 13:

- **Initial Dose**: Typically starts at **25 mg once daily** for the first 2 weeks.
- **Maintenance Dose**: Gradually increased to **100-500 mg daily** based on individual response and tolerability. The usual maintenance dose is around **300 mg/day** for most patients.

Children (Ages 2 to 12):

- **Initial Dose**: Generally starts at **0.3 mg/kg** once daily, adjusted based on weight.
- **Maintenance Dose**: Varies based on weight, typically ranging from **1-15 mg/kg/day**.

Bipolar Disorder:

Adults:

- **Initial Dose**: Starts at **25 mg once daily** for the first 2 weeks.
- **Maintenance Dose**: Usually adjusted to between **100-200 mg daily** for mood stabilization.

Important Considerations:

- **Dosage Adjustments**: Doses are often adjusted based on whether the patient is on enzyme-inducing or enzyme-inhibiting medications.
- **Titration**: It's crucial to titrate (increase the dose) slowly to minimize the risk of skin rashes and other side effects.

- **Formulations**: Lamictal is available in several formulations, including standard tablets, chewable tablets, and orally disintegrating tablets, which can influence dosing strategies.

Monitoring:

Patients should have regular follow-ups with their healthcare provider to monitor effectiveness and any side effects, especially during the initial treatment phase or when changing dosages.

Epilepsy Dosages:

Adults and Adolescents (13 years and older):

- **Initial Dose**:
    - **25 mg once daily** for the first 2 weeks.
- **Titration**:
    - After the initial 2 weeks, the dose is typically increased by **25 mg to 50**

mg every 1 to 2 weeks, depending on individual tolerance and response.

- **Maintenance Dose**:
    - The usual maintenance range is **100-500 mg per day**, with **300 mg/day** being common for many patients.
    - **Maximum Dose**: The maximum recommended dose is **500 mg/day**.

Children (Ages 2 to 12):

- **Initial Dose**:
    - **0.3 mg/kg once daily** for the first 2 weeks (with a maximum of **25 mg** for children weighing less than 25 kg).
- **Titration**:
    - Increase the dose by **0.3-0.6 mg/kg** weekly, based on clinical response and tolerability.
- **Maintenance Dose**:
    - Typically ranges from **1-15 mg/kg/day**, adjusted according to

weight. For children weighing more than 25 kg, the adult dosing guidelines may apply.

Bipolar Disorder Dosages:

Adults:

- **Initial Dose**:
    - **25 mg once daily** for the first 2 weeks.
- **Titration**:
    - Increase by **25 mg to 50 mg** every 1 to 2 weeks based on clinical response.
- **Maintenance Dose**:
    - The usual range is **100-200 mg/day**, with some patients requiring doses up to **400 mg/day** for adequate mood stabilization.

Specific Considerations:

Renal or Hepatic Impairment:

- Dosage adjustments may be necessary in patients with significant renal or liver impairment. Regular monitoring is essential.

Drug Interactions:

- **Enzyme-Inducing Drugs**: If taken with drugs that induce hepatic enzymes (e.g., carbamazepine, phenytoin), higher doses of Lamictal may be required to maintain therapeutic levels.
- **Enzyme-Inhibiting Drugs**: If taken with valproate or other enzyme inhibitors, Lamictal levels may increase, necessitating a reduction in dose.

Pregnancy and Lactation:

- Lamictal can be used during pregnancy, but dosage adjustments may be required due to hormonal changes affecting metabolism. It is also excreted in breast milk, so a careful assessment of risks and benefits is essential.

Discontinuation:

- When discontinuing Lamictal, it's important to taper the dose gradually to avoid withdrawal symptoms or increased seizure frequency.

Patient Monitoring:

- Regular follow-ups are critical, especially during the initiation of therapy and when adjusting dosages. Monitoring should include assessments of seizure frequency, mood stability, and any adverse effects, particularly skin rashes.

Lamictal is a versatile medication with dosing tailored to individual patient needs. Always consult a healthcare provider for personalized recommendations and adjustments based on response and any potential interactions.

Always consult a healthcare provider for personalized dosing recommendations tailored to individual health needs and circumstances.

CHAPTER SIX

FAQ

Frequently Asked Questions (FAQ) about Lamictal

What is Lamictal used for?

Lamictal is primarily used to treat epilepsy and bipolar disorder. In epilepsy, it helps manage partial and generalized seizures. In bipolar disorder, it is effective in stabilizing mood and managing depressive episodes.

How does Lamictal work?

Lamictal works by stabilizing neuronal membranes and inhibiting the release of excitatory neurotransmitters, which helps prevent seizures and mood episodes.

What are the common side effects of Lamictal?

Common side effects include dizziness, headache, nausea, drowsiness, insomnia, and skin rash. It's important to monitor for any serious skin reactions.

Can I take Lamictal with other medications?

Lamictal can interact with various medications, including other antiepileptic drugs, hormonal contraceptives, and some antidepressants. Always inform your healthcare provider about all medications and supplements you are taking.

How should I take Lamictal?

Lamictal is usually taken once or twice daily, with or without food. Follow your healthcare provider's instructions regarding dosage and timing. It's important to take it consistently at the same times each day.

What should I do if I miss a dose?

If you miss a dose, take it as soon as you remember. If it's close to the time for your next dose, skip the missed dose and continue with your regular schedule. Do not double the dose.

Can I stop taking Lamictal suddenly?

No, stopping Lamictal suddenly can lead to increased seizure frequency or withdrawal symptoms. If you need to discontinue the medication, consult your healthcare provider for a tapering plan.

Is Lamictal safe during pregnancy?

Lamictal can be used during pregnancy, but it's essential to discuss the potential risks and benefits with your healthcare provider, as dosage adjustments may be needed.

How long does it take for Lamictal to work?

The effectiveness of Lamictal can vary by individual and condition. It may take several weeks to notice significant improvements in mood stabilization or seizure control.

What should I do if I experience a rash?

If you develop a rash while taking Lamictal, contact your healthcare provider immediately. Rashes can indicate serious conditions, including Stevens-Johnson syndrome.

Are there any dietary restrictions while taking Lamictal?

There are no specific dietary restrictions while taking Lamictal, but it's best to discuss any dietary concerns with your healthcare provider.

Can Lamictal affect my mood?

While Lamictal is used to stabilize mood in bipolar disorder, some individuals may experience mood changes or worsening depression. Regular monitoring is essential.

If you have any additional questions or concerns about Lamictal, it's important to consult your healthcare provider for personalized advice and guidance.

www.ingramcontent.com/pod-product-compliance
Lightning Source LLC
Chambersburg PA
CBHW070959220526
45471CB00007B/3102